MIRA MAMMA

BREASTFEEDING 101

Facts and Tips to Confidently Breastfeed your Baby

First edition

This book was professionally typeset on Reedsy.
Find out more at reedsy.com

Contents

I

BREASTFEEDING 101

BREASTFEEDING is nature's intricate dance between mother and child, a timeless bond forged through nourishment and love. Yet, for many new mothers, the steps of this dance can feel unfamiliar and daunting.

In **"BREASTFEEDING 101"**, you get expert guidance, reassuring facts, and empowering tips to confidently navigate the journey of nurturing your baby and to a fulfilling breastfeeding experience.

1

INTRODUCTION

Congratulations! Whether you're an expecting mother, brand-new parent, or just someone seeking more knowledge about the marvel of breastfeeding, this book is a must-have. The journey of motherhood, sprinkled with joy, love, and challenges, often leaves parents awash with questions, and among them, the act of breastfeeding itself. Did you know that a mother's body starts preparing for breastfeeding during pregnancy, with the body producing colostrum- the baby's first food? This book seeks to unfold the myriad layers of breastfeeding, each chapter carefully crafted to enlighten, comfort, and empower you, mom.

2

BENEFITS OF BREASTFEEDING

B ... *Best for babies*

  R ... *Reduces the incidence of allergies*

  E ... *Economical*

  A ... *Antibodies rich*

  S ... *Sterile and pure*

  T ... *Temperature is always ideal*

  F ... *Fresh*

  E ... *Easy once established*

  E ... *Emotional bonding*

  D ... *Digested easily*

  I ... *Immediately available*

  N ... *Nutritionally optimal*

  G ... *Gastroenteritis greatly reduced*

Dive deep into the symbiotic relationship of breastfeeding. This is why the World Health Organization recommends breastfeeding exclusively for the first six months. Not only does it provide unparalleled nutrition for the baby, but breastfeeding can also play a role in postpartum weight loss for mothers.

BENEFITS FOR THE MOTHER AND CHILD

Fact: For the mother, breastfeeding can help burn extra calories and can reduce the risk of certain cancers.

Fact: For the baby, breastfeeding provides all the nutrients and antibodies they need.

Tip: Regular breastfeeding can also help delay the return of menstruation.

Benefits for the Mother:

1.*Uterine Contraction:* releases the hormone oxytocin, which helps the uterus return to its pre-pregnancy size faster and can reduce post-delivery bleeding.

2.*Weight Loss:* breastfeeding mothers experience more rapid postpartum weight loss due to the extra calories expended.

3.*Lower Risk of Diseases:* shown to reduce the mother's risk of breast and ovarian cancer, type 2 diabetes, and postpartum depression.

4.*Cost-effective:* breastfeeding is free, while formula and its associated supplies can be quite expensive.

5.*Convenient:* no need to prepare bottles, and breast milk is always at the right temperature.

6.*Bonding:* fosters a strong emotional bond between mother and infant.

7.*Natural Contraception:* while not entirely foolproof, exclusive breastfeeding can delay the return of menstrual cycles, acting as a form of natural birth control in the initial postpartum months.

Benefits for the Baby:

1.*Optimal Nutrition:* provides the ideal balance of nutrients for the baby, tailored to the baby's specific needs.

2.*Immunity Boost:* contains antibodies that help the baby fight off viruses and bacteria, reducing the risk of infections.

3.**Digestion:** breastmilk is easier for babies to digest compared to formula.

4.**Lower Risk of Disease:** has been linked to lower risk of asthma, allergies, ear infections, respiratory illnesses, and bouts of diarrhea in the baby.

5.**Healthy weight:** breast-fed babies are more likely to have a healthy weight as they grow, and they also face a lower risk of childhood obesity.

6.**Bonding:** physical closeness, skin-to-skin touch, and eye contact during breastfeeding help strengthen the mother-baby bond.

7.**Brain Development:** some studies suggest that breast-fed babies have better cognitive outcomes later in life.

It's important to note that while breastfeeding offers many advantages, not all mothers can or choose to breastfeed, and they should be supported in their decision. The most important thing is that the baby is fed, loved, and cared for, whether it's through breast milk, formula, or a combination of both.

3

PREPARING FOR BREASTFEEDING

Breastfeeding is a beautiful and natural process, but it can also be challenging for some new moms. Proper preparation can make a significant difference in the experience.

Here's a simple guide to help new mothers prepare for breastfeeding in terms of mind, body, and environment:

Fact: In many cultures, communities set up "breastfeeding corners" in public areas to provide a conducive environment for nursing mothers.

Tips:

·*Latch is Key:* A proper latch ensures the bay gets enough milk and prevents sore nipples.

·*Feed on Demand:* Rather than a strict schedule, feed your baby when they show signs of hunger. This also helps establish a good milk supply.

·*Trust Your Body:* Doubting whether you're producing enough milk is common, but remember, mother's bodies are designed for this. If the baby is gaining weight and producing wet diapers, you're on the right track.

·*Seek Help if Needed:* Don't hesitate to reach out to lactation consultants, pediatricians, or experienced mothers if you have concerns.

1.MIND

Educate Yourself: Read books, watch videos, or attend prenatal classes to learn about breastfeeding basics, different latch techniques, and common challenges.

Set Realistic Expectations: Every mother and baby duo are unique. Some might find breastfeeding easy, while others may face challenges. Being prepared for potential hurdles can lessen anxiety.

Seek Support: Consider joining a local or online breastfeeding support group. Sharing experiences and concerns with other moms can be incredibly reassuring.

Stay Positive: A positive mindset can help overcome minor hiccups in the journey.

Fact: A study showed that moms who had a strong intention to breast-feed were more likely to succeed, even when they faced challenges.

2.BODY

Healthy Diet: Eating a balanced diet ensures that you're getting all the essential nutrients, which will be passed on to the baby. Stay hydrated, too.

Breast Care: Use a mild, non-perfumed soap to clean your breasts. Avoiding strong soaps can prevent the nipples from becoming dry and cracked.

Practice: Familiarize yourself with different breastfeeding positions.

Rest: Sleep is essential. A well-rested mom can cope better with challenges.

Fact: The composition of breast milk changes throughout the day, with studies suggesting that evening milk might contain components that help babies sleep.

3.ENVIRONMENT

Comfortable Spot: Designate a comfortable breastfeeding area in your home. A comfy chair, a nursing pillow, and some soothing music can be helpful.

Breastfeeding Kit: Keep essentials like water, snacks, breast pads, and perhaps a book or remote control close by.

Dress for Success: Wear comfortable clothing, preferably with easy access for breastfeeding.

Limit Distractions: While it's a great time to bond with your baby, having a calm environment can make it easier, especially in the early days.

Remember, breastfeeding is a personal journey, and what works for one might not work for another. The key is to stay informed, be patient, and seek support when needed.

4

LATCHING TECHNIQUES AND HOLDING POSITIONS

The art and science of breastfeeding, demystified! Learn the secrets to achieving a comfortable and effective latch and explore various holding positions that ensure both you and your baby are relaxed.

Latch on: It's vital for efficient milk transfer and reducing nipple pain.

   Tip: Ensure baby's mouth covers a large part of the areola and not just the nipple.

PROPER LATCH ON

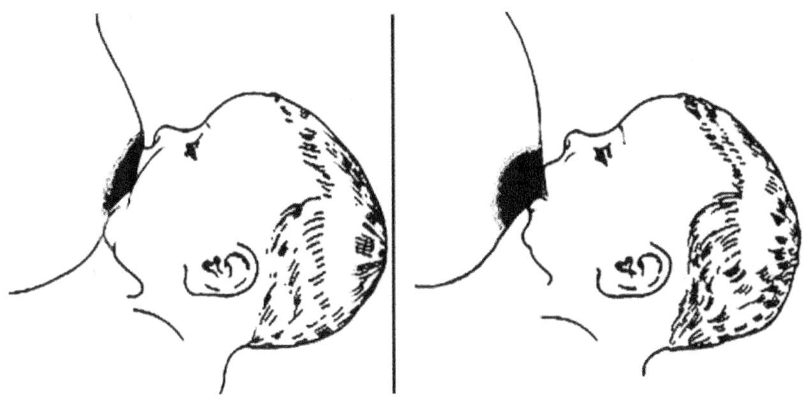

Good Attachment Bad Attachment

A proper latch means the baby's mouth covers a large portion of the areola (the dark area around the nipple) and not just the nipple itself. This ensures that the baby gets enough milk and minimizes discomfort for the mom.

STEPS TO ACHIEVE A PROPER LATCH:

1.**Mouth Wide Open:** Wait for your baby to open their mouth wide. You can encourage this by brushing your nipple against their lips.

2.**Bring Baby to Breast:** Instead of leaning down into the baby, bring the baby to your breast. Use one hand to support your baby's head and the other to hold your breast.

3.**Nipple Towards Roof of Mouth:** As you bring the baby to your breast, aim your nipple towards the roof of their mouth.

4.**Chin and Nose Touching Breast:** The baby's chin should touch your breast first, with their nose free or just barely touching the breast.

5.**Check the Latch:** Once latched, the baby's lips should be flanged out (like a fish), and you should see more of the areola above the baby's lip than below. It shouldn't feel painful to you. If it does, gently break the suction (by inserting your finger in the corner of the baby's mouth) and try again.

If the baby is well attached, the baby is probably suckling well and getting breastmilk during the feed. These signs will tell you that the baby is "drinking in the milk" and is effectively suckling:

·Slow deep sucks sometimes with short pause.
   ·May hear or see the baby swallowing.
   ·Baby's cheek is full during a feed.
   ·Baby finishes the feed and releases the breast.
   ·Looks contented.

However, these are signs that suckling is ineffective, and the baby is not getting the milk easily. Even one of these signs indicates that there may be a difficulty.

·Makes rapid shallow sucks.
   ·Makes smacking or clicking sounds.
   ·Has cheeks drawn in.
   ·Fusses or appears unsettled at the breast and comes on and off the breast.
   ·Feeds very frequently.
   ·Feeds for a long time (unless low birth weight).
   ·Not contented at the end of the feed.

HOLDING POSITIONS IN BREASTFEEDING

Breastfeeding can be a beautiful bonding experience, but it's also a skill that both mom and baby need to learn. Ensuring a proper latch and finding a comfortable holding position is essential for successful breastfeeding.

Holding Positions: Popular positions include the cradle, cross-cradle, football, and side-lying.

   Tip: Rotate positions to ensure all milk ducts get emptied, reducing the risk of mastitis.

Here's a brief rundown of popular breastfeeding positions.

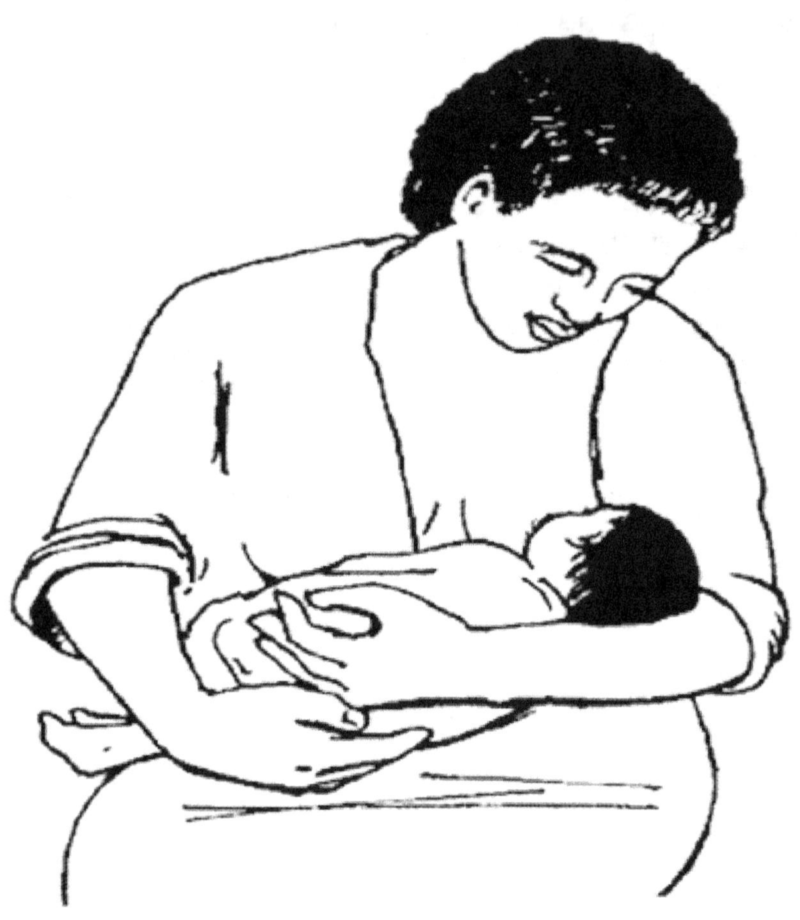

Cradle Hold:

- Sit comfortably with support pillows if needed.
- Place your baby's head in the crook of your arm (same side as the breast you're feeding from).
- Your baby's body should be facing yours, with their belly touching

your belly.

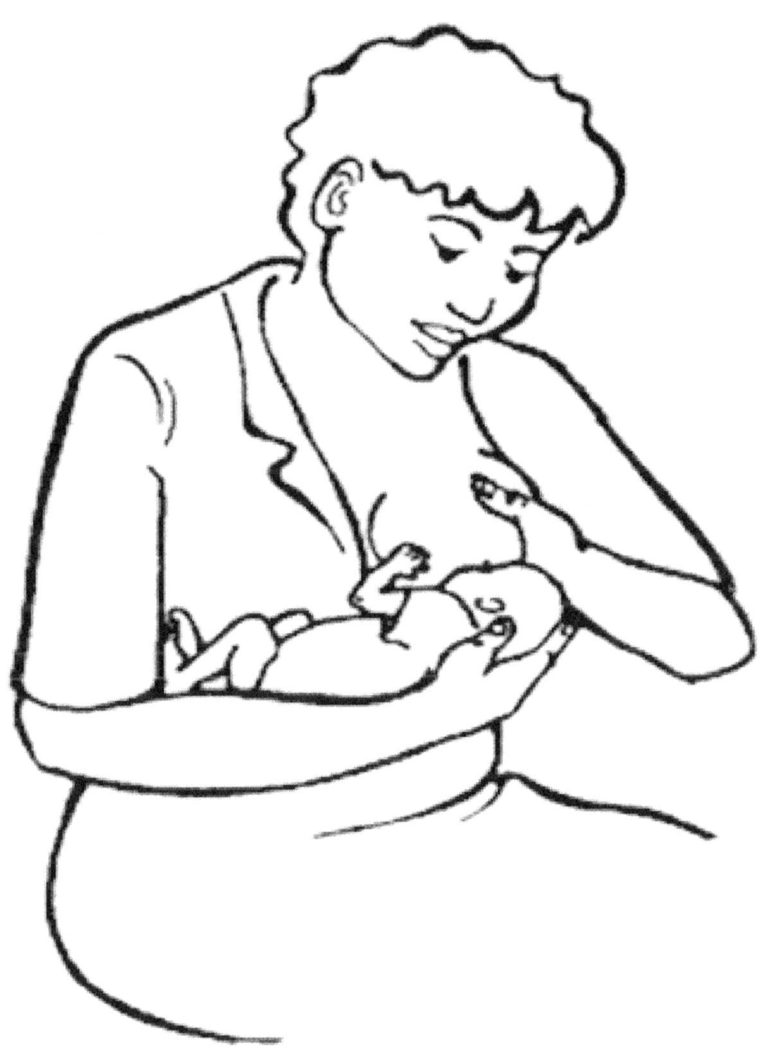

Cross-Cradle Hold:

- Similar to the cradle hold, but you'll support your baby's head with the opposite hand.
- If feeding from the right breast, use your left hand to support the baby's head and vice versa.

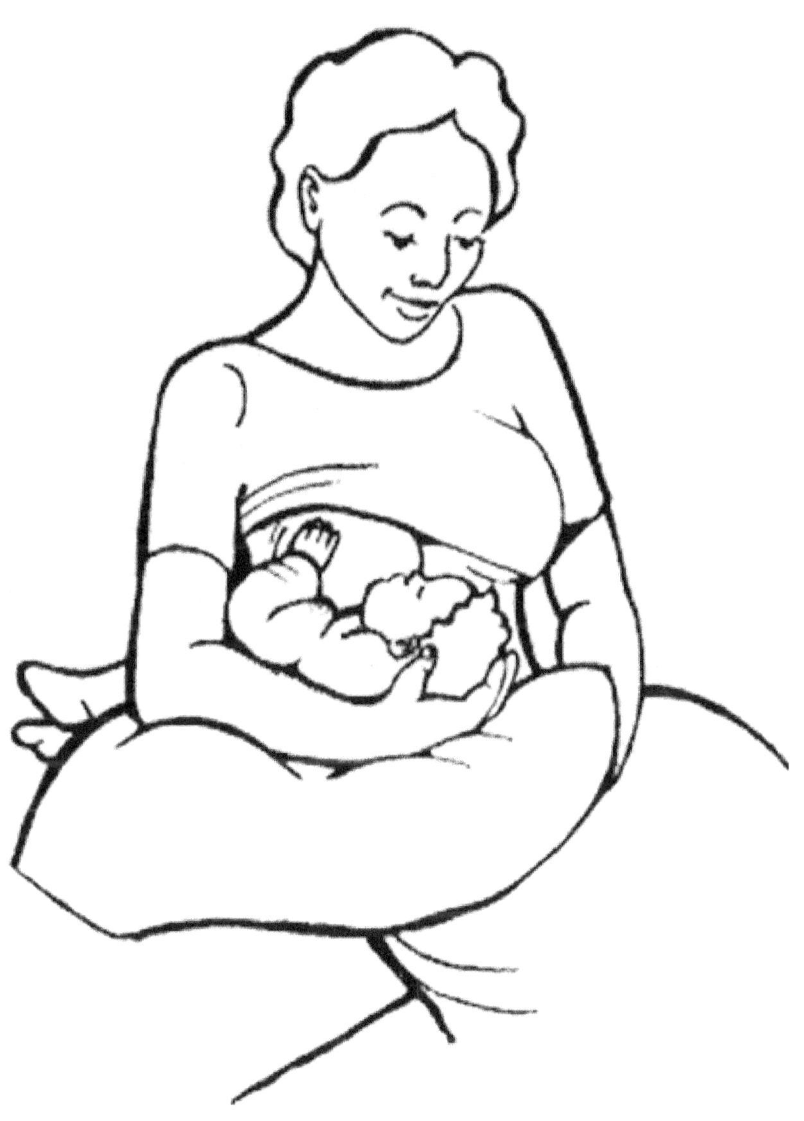

Football or Clutch Hold:

- Ideal for mothers who had a C-section.
- Hold your baby at your side, under your arm, like how you would hold a football.
- Your baby's feet and legs will be extending behind you.

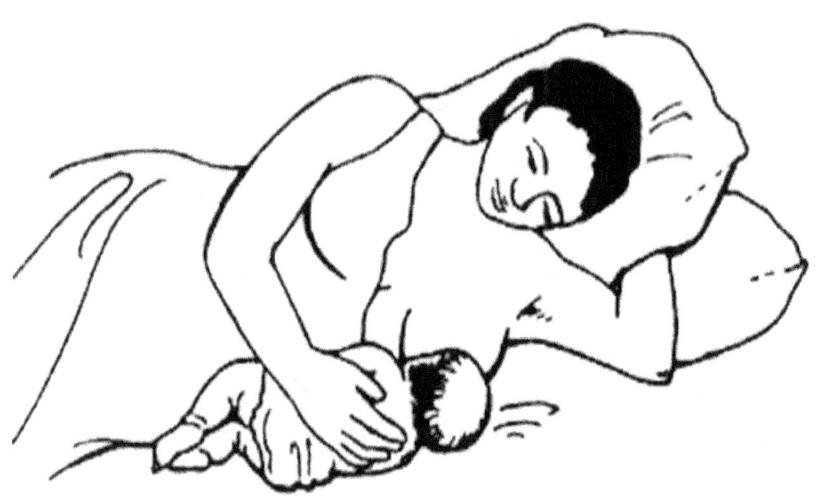

Side-Lying Position:

- Both you and your baby lie on your sides, facing each other.
- Use your arm or a pillow to support your baby's back.
- Great for nighttime feeds or if you've had a C-section.

Remember, every mom and baby duo are unique. It might take a few

tries to figure out what latch technique and position work best for you both. It's okay to ask for help and seek guidance from lactation consultants or experienced moms. The key is patience, persistence, and ensuring both you and the baby are comfortable.

5

BREASTFEEDING CHALLENGES AND DIFFICULTIES

Breastfeeding, while a natural process, can sometimes come with challenges.

From **Pain** and **Discomfort** to **Latching Problems** and **Supply Issues**, this section will guide you through potential challenges, offering solutions and solace, ensuring you're never alone in your journey.

PAIN AND DISCOMFORT DURING BREASTFEEDING

Pain and Discomfort: Some discomfort is typical but severe pain isn't.
  Tip: Ensure correct latch and use nipple cream for relief.

·**Correct Latch:** Ensure the baby's mouth covers a good portion of the areola, not just the nipple. A poor latch is a common cause of pain.
  ·**Nipple Care:** Use purified lanolin or breast milk to moisturize and heal sore nipples after feeding. Air-dry nipples after each feeding.
  ·**Breast Care:** If you have engorged breasts (very full and painful),

apply cold compresses, and express some milk to relieve pressure. Warm compresses can help with let-down and unblock milk ducts.

·**Mastitis:** This is a breast infection that can cause pain, redness, and flu-like symptoms. If you suspect mastitis, see a healthcare professional as antibiotics might be required.

·**Seek Help:** Consult a lactation consultant or breastfeeding specialist if pain persists.

LATCHING PROBLEMS DURING BREASTFEEDING

Latching Problems: Babies might struggle to latch due to various reasons.

Tip: Try different positions or seek help from a lactation consultant.

·**Breastfeeding Positions:** Experiment with different positions like the cradle, football, side-lying to find what's most comfortable.

·**Encourage Wide Mouth:** Wait for your baby to open their mouth wide, then bring them onto the breast, ensuring they take a large mouthful of the breast tissue.

·**Check for Tongue-tie:** Some babies have a condition where the tissue connecting the tongue to the floor of the mouth is too short. This can interfere with latching. A simple procedure (surgical cut) can correct this.

·**Nipple Shields:** If you have flat or inverted nipples, a silicone nipple shield might help. Always consult with a lactation consultant before using it.

·**Skin-to-skin contact:** This can help babies to instinctively seek the breast and latch.

·**Professional Guidance:** A lactation consultant or pediatrician can provide hands-on help with latching issues.

BREASTMILK SUPPLY ISSUES DURING BREASTFEEDING

Supply Issues: Some moms might feel that they aren't producing enough milk.

Tip: Feed on demand, ensure proper latch, and stay hydrated to boost supply.

·**Frequent Feedings:** The more you nurse, the more milk you produce. Feed on demand and avoid long gaps.

·**Ensure Good Latch:** A good latch ensures efficient milk transfer.

·**Breast Compression:** Gently squeezing the breast while feeding can encourage more milk to flow.

·**Stay Hydrated:** Drink plenty of water and fluids to support milk production.

·**Eat a Balanced Diet:** Nutrition plays a role in milk production. Eat a diet rich in whole grains, protein, fruits, and vegetables.

·**Limit or Avoid Pacifiers:** Early use of pacifiers can interfere with breastfeeding and reduce stimulation to produce milk.

·**Avoid Alcohol and Caffeine:** Both can reduce milk supply. Moderate caffeine is typically okay, but excessive amounts can be problematic.

·**Rest:** Fatigue can impact milk supply. Try to get as much rest as possible.

·**Medications and Herbs:** Some medications and herbs, fenugreek, blessed thistle, and others, might increase milk supply. Always check with a healthcare provider before stating any new supplements or medications.

·**Pumping:** If you're separated from your baby or if they're not feeding well, pump regularly to maintain and increase supply.

·**Reach out for Help:** If you're concerned about your supply, it's important to see a lactation consultant or healthcare provider.

Remember, every mother and baby pair are unique, and what works for one may not work for another. It's essential to stay patient and be open to trying different strategies to see what's most effective for you and your baby.

6

BREASTFEEDING HEALTH ISSUES

Breastfeeding, while often a beneficial process, can come with challenges.

Here are some common health issues associated with breastfeeding, along with simple relief and management strategies:

1.MASTITIS

Description: Inflammation of breast tissue that can result in infection. Symptoms may include redness, swelling, pain, and flu-like symptoms such as fever and chills.

Relief and Management:
·Continue breastfeeding or pumping to empty the breast.
·Apply warm compresses to the affected area.
·Massage the breast gently from the chest wall toward the nipple during nursing or pumping.
·Rest and stay hydrated.

·Wear supportive, well-fitting bras, and avoid underwires.

·If symptoms don't improve within 24 hours, or if you develop a fever, consult a healthcare provider. Antibiotics may be required.

2.ENGORGEMENT

Description: This is when the breasts become overly full of milk, leading to hardening, pain, and swelling. This commonly occurs in the first few days after birth but can happen at other times.

Relief and Management:
·Nurse your baby frequently.

·Before breastfeeding, apply warm compresses for a few minutes or take a warm shower to help milk flow.

·Apply cold packs or cold cabbage leaves after nursing to reduce swelling.

·Hand express or pump just enough to relieve discomfort.

·Wear supportive bras.

3.CRACKED OR SORE NIPPLES

Description: Tenderness or pain in the nipples, which can be caused by various factors such as improper latch, dry skin, or infection.

Relief and Management:
·Ensure your baby has a proper latch.

·Apply pure lanolin or breastmilk on the nipples after feeding.

·Allow nipples to air dry after each feeding.

·Use hydrogel pads for soothing.

·If pain persists, consider meeting with a lactation consultant.

4.BLOCKED DUCTS

Description: This happens when milk is not draining properly from a part of the breast, leading to a hard lump and soreness.

Relief and Management:
·Nurse frequently and vary breastfeeding positions.
·Apply warm compresses and massage the lump gently.
·Avoid tight bras or clothes that may constrict milk flow.

5.THRUSH (YEAST INFECTION)

Description: A fungal infection that can develop on the nipples and in the baby's mouth. Symptoms include itchy, pink, and burning nipples and a shiny or flaky skin on the nipple/areola.

Relief and Management:
·Keep nipples dry and exposed to air when possible.
·Apply antifungal creams as prescribed by a healthcare provider.
·Both mother and baby may need treatment to prevent reinfection.
·Wash hands frequently and sterilize anything that comes in contact with the baby's mouth or your nipples.

If you experience persistent problems, it's crucial to consult a health-care professional or lactation consultant. They can provide specific guidance tailored to your situation.

7

TRACKING BABY'S INTAKE AND GROWTH

Tracking the well-being of a breast-fed newborn is crucial to ensuring they are getting the nutrition and care they need.

Did you know a well-fed baby can have 6 or more wet diapers a day? Learn about **Diaper Output** and **Weight Gain Pattern** to ensure your baby's growth is on the right track.

Diaper Output: 6-8 wet diapers a day can indicate sufficient intake.
   Tip: Track diaper changes in the early weeks to gauge milk intake.

Weight Gain Pattern: Babies typically regain birth weight by 10-14 days.
   Tip: Regular pediatrician visits will monitor and track weight gain.

FREQUENCY OF BREASTFEEDING

First 24 hours: It's typical for newborns to breastfeed 1-3 times in the first day of life. They are mostly consuming colostrum during this time, which is a thick, yellowish fluid that's packed with nutrients and antibodies.

Days 2-4: Your baby might feed around 8-12 times or more in 24 hours. This helps stimulate milk production.

After the first week: A well-fed breastfed baby will typically nurse around 8-12 times in 24 hours. Some might feed even more often. This frequency helps to establish and maintain the mother's milk supply. Every baby is different, and some may have longer stretches between feedings than others, especially at night.

WET DIAPERS

Day 1: Expect about 1 wet diaper.

Day 2: Expect at least 2 wet diapers in 24 hours.

Day 3: Expect at least 3 wet diapers in 24 hours.

Day 4 and beyond: By day 4, your baby should have at least 6 or more wet diapers every 24 hours. This indicates they are getting enough milk. The urine should be pale and mild smelling.

STOOL PATTERN

First days: Babies will pass meconium, which is a sticky, black or greenish stool.

Days 3-4: The stool will transition to a greenish color.

Day 5 and beyond: Expect at least 3-4 stools daily, which should be soft and yellow. After a few weeks, the frequency might decrease, and some breastfed babies might only have a stool once a week, which can also be normal.

WEIGHT GAIN PATTERN

Initial weight loss: It's typical for newborns to lose some of their birth weight in the first few days. A loss of 5-7% is standard, but a loss of 10% or more can be concerning.

Regaining weight: By day 5-7, babies should start gaining weight. By about two weeks, most babies will have regained their birth weight or even surpassed it.

Continued growth: After regaining their birth weight, a typical weight gain for a breastfed baby is about 4-7 ounces (110-200 grams) per week for the first few months.

Remember, every baby is unique, and what's normal for one might be different for another. It's essential to work closely with a pediatrician to ensure that your baby's growth and feeding patterns are on track. If there are concerns about breastfeeding, weight gain, or anything else, seek guidance from a lactation consultant or a healthcare professional.

8

WEANING AND TRANSITION TO SOLID FOOD

Determining when your baby is ready for weaning and introducing them to solid foods is an exciting and significant milestone.

As your little one grows, the dance of **Gradual Weaning** and the excitement of **Introducing Solid Foods** await. Discover how to make this transition smooth and enjoyable.

Gradual Weaning Techniques: Dropping one feeding at a time reduces discomfort.
  Tip: Offer a sippy cup during missed feeding times.

Introducing Solid Foods: Usually starts around 6 months.
  Tip: Start with single-ingredient foods and monitor for allergies.

SIGNS YOUR BABY IS READY TO BE WEANED

Although every baby is different, most babies are ready to start weaning around 6 months of age. Before this time, breastmilk or formula provides all the nutrients a baby needs. Look for these signs:

1.**Holding Head Up:** Your baby should be able to hold their head up and sit up straight with some support.

2.**Hand-to-Mouth Coordination:** Your baby starts putting things into their mouth and may try to grab what you're eating.

3.**Swallowing Skills:** If you give your baby a little solid food or puree, they won't just push it out of their mouth with their tongue.

4.**Increased Appetite:** Even after a full milk feed, your baby still seems hungry.

5.**Curiosity about Food:** Your baby shows interest in your food, looking at what you're eating, and may even reach for it.

GRADUAL WEANING TECHNIQUES

It's important to take a slow approach:

1.**Start with Single Ingredient: Initially, introduce one food at a time. This helps in identifying any allergies or intolerances.**

2.**Start Small: Begin with a few spoonsful of a single-ingredient puree, mashed fruit, or well-cooked, mashed veggies.**

3. **Introduce a Sippy Cup:** Around 6 months, you can introduce a sippy cup with water during meals.

4. **Mix with Familiar:** To make new foods more palatable, you can mix them with breast milk or formula.

5.**Monitor for Allergies:** After introducing a new food, wait a few days before introducing another. This helps spot potential allergic reactions, like rashes, diarrhea, or vomiting.

FIRST INTRODUCTION OF SOLID FOODS

1.Choose a Good Time: Pick a time when your baby is relaxed but slightly hungry. They shouldn't be too hungry or too full.

2.Stay with Soft Textures: Start with smooth purees like mashed bananas, apple puree, or well-cooked and mashed sweet potatoes.

3.Introduce Cereals: Baby rice or oatmeal, mixed with breastmilk or formula, can be a good start.

4.Use a Baby Spoon: Introduce a soft-tipped spoon, allowing your baby to explore and play with it.

5. Be Ready for Mess: It's a learning process, and babies are likely to spit out, play with, or drop food.

6.Follows Baby's Lead: Pay attention to cues. If they're turning away or not interested, don't push.

7.Gradually Increase Variety: Once your baby gets used to one food, introduce another. Gradually build up the textures from pureed to mashed, then finely chopped.

8.Avoid Certain Foods: Honey shouldn't be given before age 1 due to the risk of botulism. Limit high allergenic foods and always monitor when introducing them (like peanuts, tree nuts, dairy, eggs, soy, wheat, fish, and shellfish). Also, avoid giving foods that pose a choking hazard.

9.Introduce Finger Foods: Around 7-9 months, as the baby develops a pincer grip, they can be given soft finger foods like soft-cooked carrot sticks or soft fruits.

10.Stay Patient and Flexible: Your baby may love food one day and hate it the next. That's normal! The key is persistence and patience.

Always remember, during the weaning process, milk (breastmilk or formula) will still be your baby's main source of nutrition until their first birthday. Discuss your plans with a pediatrician or a child

nutritionist to ensure your baby is getting all the necessary nutrients.

9

LEGAL AND WORKPLACE ISSUES

Breastfeeding in public and managing lactation needs in the workplace can be a concern for many new mothers. Both situations require a balance between the mother's right to feed or express milk for her child and societal or organizational expectations.

Become informed and confident about your rights concerning **Breast-feeding in Public** and understand the **Workplace Policies for Nursing Mothers**. Knowledge is power, and with it, you can create a conducive environment for you and your baby.

Breastfeeding in Public: Most countries and states protect a mother's right to breastfeed in public.
   Tip: Use a cover if you're more comfortable but know your rights.

Workplace policies for Nursing Mothers: Federal law often requires employers to provide break time and a space for pumping.
   Tip: Discuss your needs and rights with HR before returning to work.

BREASTFEEDING IN PUBLIC

Know Your Rights: Many countries and regions have laws that explicitly allow women to breastfeed in any public or private location. Research local laws to know your rights.

Wear Appropriate Clothing: Many women find it easier to breastfeed discreetly by wearing tops that allow easy access or by using a nursing cover. However, the choice of how to dress and whether to cover up is entirely up to each mother.

Scout Locations: If you're uncomfortable breastfeeding openly in public, look for more secluded or quieter places. Some places like shopping malls or airports have dedicated nursing rooms.

Use a Sling or Carrier: Many baby carriers allow for discreet nursing, so you can breastfeed on-the-go.

Stay Calm: If someone confronts you, it helps to remain calm and assertive. If you know the laws, you can explain them politely.

WORKPLACE POLICIES FOR LACTATING WORKING MOMS

Break Time for Nursing Mothers: In many regions, employers are required to provide break time for mothers to express breast milk. This time may or may not be paid, depending on local labor laws.

Private Space: Employers should provide a place, other than a bathroom, shielded from view and free from intrusion, where an employee can express breast milk. This can be a dedicated lactation room or a temporary space, as long as it's available when needed.

Supportive Management: It's essential for managers and HR professionals to support lactating mothers, recognizing that the ability to express milk or nurse during working hours boosts morale and decreases time taken off work due to child illnesses.

Employee Education: Employers can offer resources or even classes about breastfeeding, which can help not only the nursing moms but also their co-workers, to create a more understanding environment.

Flexed Scheduling: If possible, employers can provide flexible scheduling for nursing moms, allowing them to either come in late, leave early, or take longer breaks to accommodate their nursing or pumping schedule.

Fridge or Cooler Access: Many women need a place to store their expressed milk safely. Providing access to a refrigerator or allowing employees to bring a small cooler can be beneficial.

Clear Policies: It's essential for employers to have a clear and written lactation policy in place. This policy should be communicated to all employees to ensure that everyone understands the rights and needs of nursing mothers.

For working moms, the return to work can be more manageable when there's an understanding of what to expect and what resources are available. Similarly, the more society becomes accustomed to seeing mothers breastfeed in public, the more normalized and accepted it will become.

10

NUTRITION AND WELLNESS FOR THE BREASTFEEDING MOTHER

Dive into the essentials of **Nutrition for Lactating Mothers**. Beyond physical health, delve into **Emotional Wellness** and nurturing your bond and **Reconnecting with your Partner**.

Nutrition for Lactating Mothers: Moms need an extra 500 calories a day.

Tip: Prioritize nutrient-dense foods and drink plenty of water.

NUTRITION FOR LACTATING MOTHERS

A well-nourished body helps to ensure an adequate supply of breast milk. Breastfeeding mothers should prioritize a balanced diet that includes:

Caloric Intake: On average, a breastfeeding mother requires an additional 300-500 calories per day. This can vary based on the mother's activity level and the baby's needs.

Proteins: Increase protein intake with foods like lean meats, eggs, dairy products, beans, and nuts.

Calcium and Vitamin D: Essential for both the mother and baby's bone health. Include dairy products, fortified foods, and leafy greens in your diet.

Omega -3 Fatty Acids: These can be found in fatty fish, flax seeds, and walnuts. They are crucial for the baby's brain development.

Iron and Zinc: Essential minerals found in meats, beans, nuts, and whole grains.

Hydration: Drink plenty of water, at least 8-10 glasses per day, to stay hydrated and support milk production.

Emotional Wellness: Postpartum emotions can be a roller coaster.
  Tip: Seek support and practice self-care regularly.

EMOTIONAL WELLNESS

Breastfeeding can be an emotional journey with its set of challenges. Here's how to maintain emotional wellness:

Rest: It's essential to sleep whenever you get a chance. Lack of sleep can contribute to mood swings and stress.

Seek Support: Talk to friends, family, or join support groups. Sharing experiences and seeking advice can provide immense relief.

Mindfulness and Relaxation: Engage in relaxation techniques like meditation, deep breathing exercises, and gentle exercise like walking or yoga.

Reach out for Professional Help: If feelings of sadness, anxiety, or depression persist, consult a therapist or counselor.

Reconnecting with Partner: Intimacy can change post-baby.

   Tip: Communicate openly with your partner about your feelings and needs.

RECONNECTING WITH PARTNER

The arrival of a baby can sometimes create distance between partners. Here's how to reconnect:

Open Communication: Share your feelings, needs, and concerns with your partner. Understand each other's roles and responsibilities.

Take Time Out Together: Even if it's just for a short while, spending quality time can help you both reconnect. This could be a simple dinner or a walk together.

Physical Intimacy: While it's common for sexual desire to decrease during the postpartum period, other forms of physical affection, such as hugging, holding hands, or cuddling, can maintain closeness.

Seek Counseling: If you both feel distant, consider couples counseling to address any underlying issues.

II

EXTRAS

11

PARTS OF THE BREAST

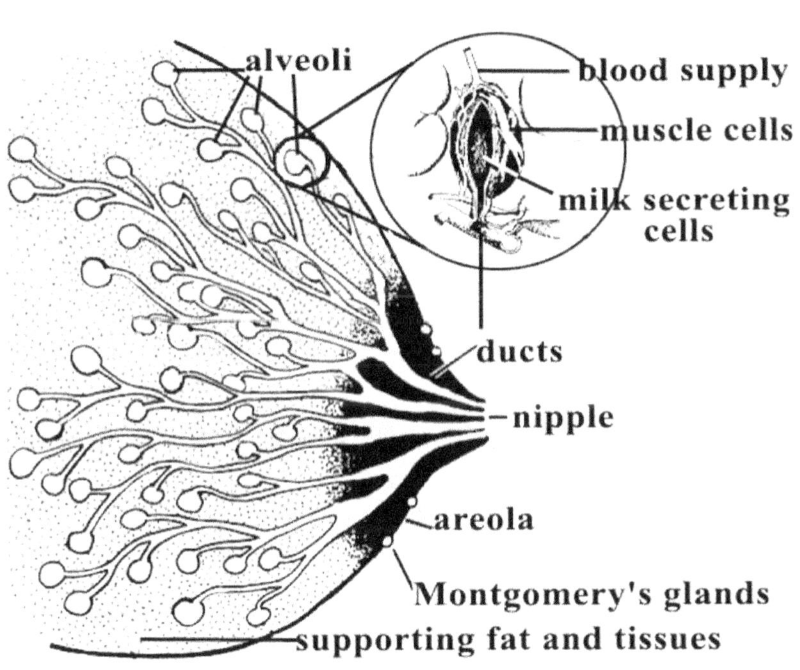

12

HOW TO SUPPORT THE BREAST

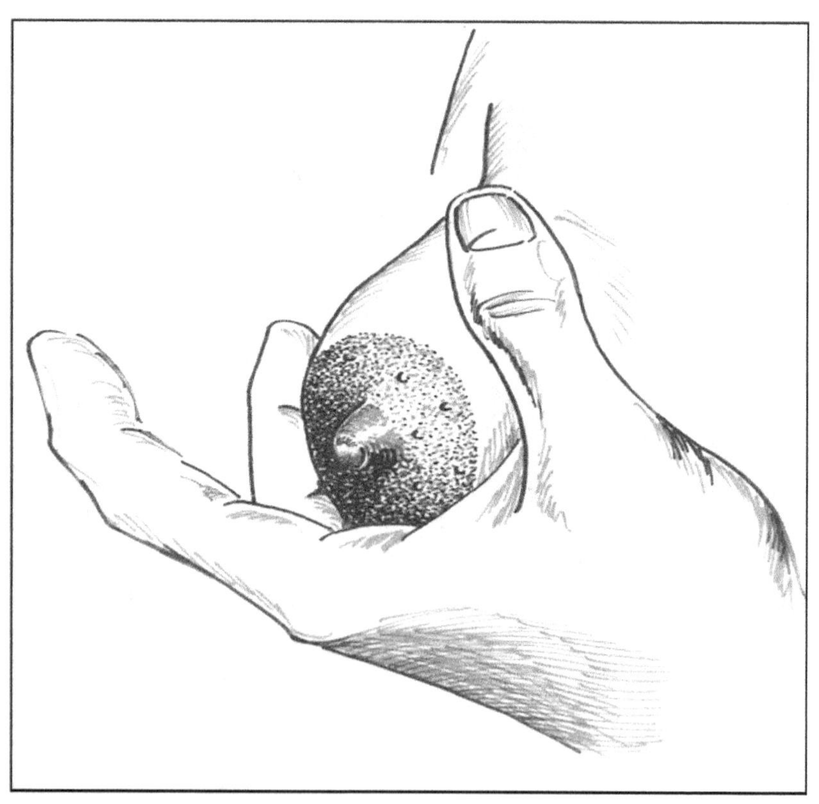

45

13

MANUAL EXPRESSION

Find the milk ducts

Gently feel the breast near the outer edge of the areola or about the length of the first thumb joint back from the nipple (ABOUT one and a half inches or 4cms) until you find a place where the breast feels different. You may describe it as feeling like a knotted string or a row of peas. These are the ducts of milk. Depending on what part of the breast it is, the mother should place her first finger over the duct, and her thumb on the opposite side of the breast, or her thumb on the duct and finger opposite. Support breast with the other fingers of that hand, or with the other hand.

Compress the breast over the ducts

Gently press the thumb and fingers slightly back towards the chest wall. Then press the thumb and first finger together, compressing the milk duct between them. This helps the milk to flow towards the nipple. Release the pressure and repeat the compress and release movement until milk starts to drip out (it may take a few minutes). Colostrum may come out in drops, as it is thick and a small amount. Later the milk may spray out in streams after the oxytocin reflex works.

Repeat in all parts of the breast

When the milk flow slows, the mother moves the thumb and finger around the edge of the areola to another section and repeats the press and release movement. When flow ceases, change to the other breast and repeat, if both breasts are to be expressed. The mother can pause to massage her breast again if needed. She can go back and forth between her breasts a few times if needed.

It takes practice to get large volumes of milk. First milk (colostrum) may only come in drops. These are precious to your baby.

How often to express depends on the reason for expressing. If your baby is very young and not feeding at the breast, you will need to express every 2-3 hours. It is important to have clean hands and clean containers for the milk.

How long to express?

The length of time to express depends on why the mother is expressing.

·To get colostrum for the baby who is not able to suck, mom might express for 5-10 minutes to get a teaspoon of colostrum. Remember the newborn baby's stomach is very small and small amounts every 1-2 hours if what the baby needs.

·To increase milk production, aim to express for about 20 minutes at least six or more times in 24 hours including at least once at night, so that the total time expressing is at least 100 minutes per 24 hours.

·If the mother is just softening the areola to help the baby attach, she may only need to compress 3 or 4 times.

·If the mother is clearing a blocked duct, she compresses and massages until the lump has cleared.

·If it is past the newborn stage and the mother is expressing milk to be given to her baby when she is at work, determine the length of time to express by the flow of milk and the amount needed to meet the baby's needs. Some mothers can get the amount of milk needed in 15 minutes and for some women it may take 30 minutes.

·A mother might express one breast and feed the baby from the other breast.

Preterm babies and some sick babies may take only very small feeds at first. Encourage small frequent feeds of colostrum. Even very small feeds may be useful - do not dismiss small amounts that the mother expresses.

Colostrum may only come in drops. These are precious to the baby. The mother may be able to express into a spoon, small cup or directly into the baby's mouth so that no drops of colostrum are lost. A useful way is for a helper to draw up the colostrum in a syringe directly from the nipple as the mother expresses it – 1 ml can look quite a lot in a small syringe.

When a woman breastfeeds a baby to whom she did not give birth, it is called **wet nursing.** Expressed milk from another mother is called **donor milk.**

Some places may have breastmilk banks to provide milk for babies who are preterm or ill. In a milk bank, the donor mothers are screened for HIV and other illnesses and the milk is also pasteurized (heat-treated). Using donor-banked milk is usually a short-term option, as the supply may be limited, and another way of feeding will need to be discussed.

14

CUP FEEDING

Cup feeding can be used for babies who are able to swallow but cannot (yet) suckle well enough to feed themselves fully from the breast. They may have difficulty attaching well, or they may attach and suckle for a short time, but tire quickly before they have obtained enough milk. A baby of 30-32 weeks gestation can often begin to take feed from a cup.

If a baby takes a small feed, offer the next feed a little earlier, especially if the baby shows signs of hunger.

A cup does not need to be sterilized in the same way as a bottle and teat. It has an open, smooth surface that is easy to clean by washing it in hot soapy water. Avoid tight spouts, lids, or rough surfaces where milk may stick and allow bacteria to grow.

Advantages of Cup Feeding

·It is pleasant for the baby – there are no invasive tubes in his or her mouth.

·It allows the baby to use his or her tongue and to learn tastes.

·It stimulates the baby's digestion.

·It encourages coordinated breathing/suck/swallow.

·The baby needs to be held close and eye-contact is possible.

·It can allow the baby to control the amount and rate of feeding.

·A cup is easier to keep clean than a bottle and teat.

·It may be seen as a transitional method on the way to breastfeeding rather than as a 'failure' of breastfeeding.

15

STORING EXPRESSED BREASTMILK

·Choose a suitable container made of glass or plastic that can be kept covered. Clean it by washing it in hot soapy water and rinsing in hot clear water. If the mother is hand expressing, she can express directly into the container.

·If storing several containers, each container should be labeled with the date. Use the oldest milk first.

·The baby should consume expressed milk as soon as possible after expression. Feeding fresh milk (rather than frozen) is encouraged.

·Frozen breastmilk may be thawed slowly in a refrigerator and used within 24 hours. It can be defrosted by standing in a jug of warm water and used within one hour, as it is warm. Do not boil milk or heat it in a microwave as this destroys some of its properties and can burn the baby's mouth.

<u>Fresh Milk</u>

At 25-37 degrees Celsius for 4 hours,

at 15-25 degrees Celsius for 8 hours,

below 15 degrees Celsius for 24 hours.

Milk should not be stored above 37 degrees Celsius.

Refrigerated (2-40 degrees Celsius): up to 8 days.

Place the container of milk in the coldest part of the refrigerator or freezer. Many refrigerators do not keep a constant temperature. Thus, a mother may prefer to use milk within 3-5 days or freeze milk that will not be used within 5 days, if she has a freezer.

Frozen Milk

In a freezer compartment inside refrigerator: 2 weeks

In a freezer part of a refrigerator-freezer: 3 months

In a separate deep freeze: 6 months

Thawed in a refrigerator: 24 hours (do not re-freeze) or place the container in warm water to thaw quickly.

III

JOURNAL YOUR BREASTFEEDING JOURNEY

The road of breastfeeding is better traveled with company. Find out about Support Groups, Online Forums and Social Media Groups you can share, learn, and grow with fellow mothers.

Always remember that while these online platforms are wonderful sources of information and emotional support, it's also essential to consult professionals like lactation consultants or pediatricians if you have specific concerns or challenges with breastfeeding.

IV

CONCLUSION

Embrace every drop of knowledge and every ounce of love. With the right guidance, support, and faith in yourself, you can confidently nurture your baby, fortifying the bond that only grows stronger with time. Here's to the beautiful journey ahead, filled with love, growth, and countless precious moments with your little one.

www.ingramcontent.com/pod-product-compliance
Lightning Source LLC
Chambersburg PA
CBHW070723260726
48660CB00007B/2697